I0456104

Magical Eating

A Worldwide Guide

Emily Caprice Candler

Copyright Notice

Table of Contents

Contents

Introduction

If you are reading this book than you share my passion and interest in healthy eating. Knowing which foods are the best and worst helps balance your diet so you can make the right choices for you - no matter what your goal is. With so many restaurants to go to, looking up calorie information for every cuisine separately seemed like a daunting task - hence the idea for this guidebook. A complete worldwide guidebook designed to cover the Do's and Don'ts for 23 of the most common countries and cuisines. Whether you desire Korean food or are going on a trip to Korea – you can open the pages here to find the best and worst choices.

Each country has certain specialties that are highlighted in each section. I do not repeat myself by putting grilled chicken and vegetables in every country – they are healthy foods but this is more focused on the specific cuisine of the country listed. Some countries have more listed than others but there is enough variety so you will be able to recognize items on the menu.

That doesn't mean you have to eat only the 'Do's' all the time. With planning and knowledge you can enjoy the 'Don'ts' without feeling guilty about it. When you know that most of your meals have been healthy choices you can enjoy Belgian French Fries and any other specialty foods you are craving! Focusing on healthy choices allows you to plan for the not so healthy choices. Life is too short not to enjoy it!

Each country in the book is lined up with a Do's and Don'ts section. 'Do's' are foods that are the best choices for that country or cuisine. 'Don'ts' are the foods that are not the best choices. Each lists the food, description (if the food is not in English), calories and serving size in both American and Metric measurements. Some calories may vary depending on who cooks the dish. The calories listed are a close average of what to expect for that specific food.

This is intended to be a guidebook that you can take anywhere or reference at home. It is not intended to be a complete diet or fitness guide. There are many programs out there that can give you detailed information on fitness and nutrition. For a complete Fitness and Diet program I recommend Tom Venuto's "Burn the Fat, Feed the Muscle" Program.

Enjoy!!

Asia

China

Do's:

- Chicken and broccoli (no rice)
  - Calories: 280. Serving size (8 oz) (226 grams)

- Egg drop soup
  - Calories: 120. Serving size (8 oz) (226 grams)

- Steamed vegetables
  - Calories: 60. Serving size (8 oz) (226 grams)

- Brown Rice
  - Calories: 108. Serving size (4 oz) (113 grams)

- Meat, poultry, shellfish (grilled, steamed, broiled; lean)
  - Calories: Average 231. Serving size (8 oz) (226 grams)

- Moo Goo Gai Pan (Chicken w/ mushroom dish)
  - Calories 216. Serving size (8 oz) (226 grams)

Don'ts:

- Sweet and sour chicken
  - Calories: 400. Serving Size (4 oz) (113 grams)

- Fried rice
  - Calories: 360. Serving Size (8 oz) (226 grams)

- Dumplings
  - Calories: 280. Serving Size (5 oz) (140 grams)

- Noodles
  - Calories: 210. Serving Size (8 oz) (226 grams)

- Lo Mein
  - Calories: 320. Serving Size (8 oz) (226 grams)

- Large Egg Roll
  - Calories: 372. Serving Size (1.9 oz) (52 grams)

- Crispy duck
  - Calories: 470. Serving Size (9 oz) (255 grams)

Japanese

Do's:

- Fish Baked – (Cod, Haddock, Plaice, Sole)
  - Calories: Average 100 calories (3 oz) (85 grams)

- White Fish Sashimi (Raw Fish, no Rice)
  - Calories: 21 Calories (1 oz) (28 grams)

- Sashimi (Any Raw Fish on the Menu, no Rice)
  - Calories: From 19-57 Calories (1 oz) (28 grams)

- Sautéed Vegetables
  - Calories: 110. Serving size (5 oz) (141 grams)

- Soba Noodles
  -Calories: 113. Serving size (8 oz) (226 grams)

- Miso soup
  - Calories: 85. Serving Size (8 oz) (226 grams)

- Tofu
  - Calories: 88. Serving Size (4 oz) (113 grams)

- Edamame
  -Calories: 120. Serving Size (4 oz) (113 grams)

Don'ts:

- Fried Dumplings
  - Calorie Average: 572 (4 Dumplings)

- Tempura (Deep Fried Vegetable or Seafood)
  - Calorie Average: 508 (6 pieces)

Korean

Do's:

- Mehoontang (Hot Fish Soup)
  - Calories: 40. Serving Size (8 oz) (226 grams)

- Sollungtang (Beef & Noodles in a milky bone broth)
  - Calories: 87. Serving size (8 oz) (226 grams)

- Soondubu Chigae (Spicy Tofu Soup)
  -Calories 222. Serving Size (8 oz) (226 grams)

- Kimchi (Spicy Cabbage)
  -Calories: 20. Serving Size (3.5 oz) (100 grams)

- Tteok Boki (Rice Cakes with Eggs and Vegetables)
  -Calories: 209. Serving Size (8 oz) (226 grams)

- Bulgogi (Barbecued Beef)
  - Calories: 310. Serving Size (3.5 oz) (99 grams)

- Dwaenjang chigae (Soybean Paste Soup)
  Calories: 274. Serving Size (8 oz) (226 grams)

Don'ts:

- Bibimbap (Vegetables and Beef over Rice w/ Oil)
  - Calories: 560.6. Serving Size (8 oz) (226 grams)

- Samgyetang (Ginseng Chicken Soup w/ Skin)
  Calories: 735. Serving Size (8 oz) (226 grams)

Thai

Do's:

- Yam Talay (Seafood salad) without dressing
  - Calories: 150. Serving Size (5 oz) (142 grams)

- Larb Gai (Chicken Salad)
  - Calories: 168. Serving Size (5 oz) (142 grams)

- Nam Pla (Fish Sauce, as a sauce or dressing)
  - Calories: 19. Serving Size (0.5 oz) (14 grams)

- Tom Yum Goong (Spicy Shrimp Soup) OR Tom Yum Gai (Chicken Soup)
  - Calories: 187. Serving Size (8 oz) (226 grams)

- Chicken Satay
  - Calories: 135 Serving Size: 1 skewer (2.5 oz) (71 grams)

- Spring rolls
  - Calories: 120 Serving Size: 2 rolls (1.5 oz) (42 grams)

- Steamed dumplings
  - Calories: 46 Serving Size: 1 dumpling

- Sole Pan Fried fish w/ Lemon Butter Sauce
  - Calories: 268. Serving Size (7 oz) (198 grams)

Don'ts:

- Deep Fried Fish Balls
  - Calories: 1146. Serving Size (10 oz) (280 grams)

- Pad Thai
  - Calories: 430. Serving Size (10 oz) (280 grams)

- Curries
  - Calories: 340. Serving Size (8 oz) (226 grams)

- Peanut sauce or dressing
  - Calories: 70. Serving Size (0.5 oz) (14 grams)

- Sweet and sour sauce
  - Calories: 29. Serving Size (1 oz) (28 grams)

Indian

Do's:

- Chicken Biryani (Rice and Chicken)
  - Calories: 205 (Serving Size: (5.5 oz) (155 grams)

- Roti (Unleavened Flat Bread)
  - Calories: 60 (Serving Size: 1 piece, 7'' diameter)

- Bread Poori (Unleavened Wheat Bread of India)
  - Calories: 112 (Serving Size: 1 piece)

- Stuffed Paratha (Indian wheat unleavened bread stuffed with Vegetables)
  - Calories: 225. Serving Size (6 oz) (173 grams)

- Samosas (Potato stuffed Pastry)
  - Calories: 252. Serving Size (3.5 oz) (100 grams)

- Mutter Paneer (Curry of peas & home-made cheese cubes)
  - Calories: 160. Serving Size (5 oz) (141 grams)

- Bhindi Ki Subji (Stir-fried okra)
  - Calories: 46. Serving Size (4 oz) (118 grams)

Don'ts:

- Gaajar Ka Halwa (Carrot Pudding Dessert)
  - Calories: 432. Serving Size (7 oz) (204 grams)

- Papri Chaat (Deep Fried Potato w/ Yogurt)
  - Calories: 300. Serving Size (8 oz) (226 grams)

- Dahi Batata Puri (Puffed Puris filled w/ Potato, Yogurt, etc)
  - Calories: 565. Serving Size (8 oz) (226 grams)

- Aloo Chaat (Deep Fried Potato w/ Sauce)
  - Calories: 350. Serving Size (8 oz) (226 grams)

- Korma, Makhani (Curry Dishes)
  - Calories: 350. Serving Size (9.2 oz) (262 grams)

- Malpua or Jalebi (Funnel cake)
  - Calories: 655. Serving Size (6 oz) (170 grams)

Middle East

Turkish

Do's:

- Manti (Turkish Dumpling with Yogurt Sauce)
  - Calories: 170. Serving Size (3.5 oz) (98 grams)

- Etli Kuru Fasulye (Butter Beans with Meat)
  - Calories: 340. Serving Size (3.5 oz) (100 grams)

- Swordfish Kebabs
  - Calories: 150. Serving Size (6 oz) (170 grams)

- Kibrisli Bulgur Pilavi (Cracked Wheat Pilaf)
  - Calories: 261. Serving Size (7.3 oz) (209 grams)

- Zeytinyagli Yaprak Sarmasi (Vine Leaf Wraps with Olive Oil)
  - Calories: 40. Serving Size 1 Vine Leaf (1.5 oz) (45 grams)

- Ling Filet (Fish)
  - Calories: 125. Serving Size (7 oz) (200 grams)

Don'ts:

- Kofta (Turkish Meatballs w/ Lamb)
  - Calories: 482. Serving Size (5.5 oz) (155 grams)

- Su Boregi (Pastry w/ Cheese)
  - Calories: 672. Serving Size (10 oz) (285 grams)

- Gözleme (Crepes) (w/ Spinach and Feta listed)
  - Calories: 647. Serving Size (7.5 oz) (215 grams)

- Guvec Kebabi (Lamb Casserole)
  - Calories: 429. Serving Size (6 oz) (170 grams)

- Karniyarik (Cut-Belly Eggplants, Stuffed with Meat Filling)
  - Calories: 500. Serving Size (1 large Eggplant)

Egyptian

Do's:

- Bamya (Meat and Okra Stew)
  - Calories: 199. Serving Size (9.6 oz) (273 grams)

- Molokheya (Egyptian Spinach Soup w/ Chicken)
  - Calories: 338. Serving Size (6.7 oz) (190 grams)

- Orze Madses (Egyptian Salty Rice)
  - Calories: 175. Serving Size (4 oz) (113 grams)

- Megadarra (Brown Lentils and Rice with Caramelized Onions)
  - Calories: 222. Serving Size (4 oz) (113 grams)

- Yaprak Dolma (Stuffed Grape Leaves)
  - Calories: 35. Serving Size 1 pc (1 oz) (28 grams)

- Sahlab (Egyptian Spiced Drink - Sweet)
  - Calories: 207. Serving Size (5 oz) (139 grams)

- Koshary (Lentils and Rice)
  - Calories: 274. Serving Size (6 oz) (175 grams)

- Fig cakes (Rolled into Small Balls)
  - Calories: 150. Serving Size: (1.4 oz) (39 grams)

Don'ts:

- Egyptian Faatah (Rice & Meat With Crispy Bread on Bottom)
  - Calories: 1193. Serving Size (10.5 oz) (300 grams)

- Basbousa (Sweet Cakes w/ Syrup)
  - Calories: 327. Serving Size (4 oz) (113 grams)

- Um Ali (Pastry Dessert)
  - Calories: 491. Serving Size (7.3 oz) (208 grams)

Persian

Do's:

- Fesenjan (Walnuts, Pomegranate w/ Chicken over Rice)
  - Calories: 270. (5.5 oz) (155 grams)

- Pomegranate Molasses (Pomegranate Syrup)
  - Calories: 50. Serving Size 1 tbsp (0.5 oz) (14 grams)

- Basmati Rice with Butter
  - Calories: 194. Serving Size (6 oz) (170 grams)

- Gormeh Sabzi (Persian Stew with Lamb and Herbs)
  - Calories: 224. Serving Size (4.5 oz) (130 grams)

- Baba Ghannouj (Eggplant Dip)
  - Calories: 80. Serving Size (1 oz) (30.0 grams)

- Tas Kebab (Stew Casserole)
  - Calories: 168. Serving Size (5 oz) (140 grams)

- Haleem (mixture of wheat, lentils and meat)
  - Calories: 190. Serving Size (4 oz) (113 grams)

Don'ts:

- Halva (Rose Scented Dessert)
  - Calories: 847. Serving Size (5.7 oz) (162 grams)

- Ma'amoul (Date or Walnut Stuffed Pastry)
  - Calories: 230. Serving Size: (1.4 oz) (40 grams)

- Lokum (Turkish Delight – Lemon Candy)
  - Calories: 295. Serving Size: (3.5 oz) (100 grams)

- Sweet Tasting Baklava (Dessert)
  - Calories: 428. Serving Size (3.5 oz) (100 grams)

Israeli

Do's:

- Salat Yisraeli (Vegetable Salad)
  - Calories: 43. Serving Size (5.6 oz) (159 grams)

- Shakshuka (Tomato and Egg Dish)
  - Calories: 104. Serving Size (7 oz) (198 grams)

- Blintzes (Cheese Filled)
  - Calories: 80. Serving Size (2.1 oz) (60 grams)

- Cholent (Meat and Potato Stew)
  - Calories: 350. Serving Size (8 oz) (226 grams)

Don'ts:

- Jachnun (Slow Baked Bread)
  - Calories: 288. Serving Size (3.5 oz) (100 grams)

- Falafel (Fried Chickpea and Herb Balls)
  - Calories: 333. Serving Size (3.5 oz) (100 grams)

- Honey Cake
  - Calories: 387. Serving Size (4.5 oz) (128 grams)

Europe

Russian

Do's:

- Kefir (Milk Drink)
  - Calories: 120. Serving Size (8 oz) (226 grams)

- Golubzi (Cabbage Rolls Stuffed w/ Meat)
  - Calories: 111. Serving Size (3.5 oz) (100 grams)

- Kvass (Drink)
  - Calories: 125 Serving Size (16 oz) (453 grams)

- Chanterelle Mushrooms in Sour Cream Sauce
  - Calories: 135. Serving Size (8 oz) (226 grams)

- Borscht (Beetroot Soup)
  - Calories: 78. Serving size (8 oz) (226 grams)

- Schi (Cabbage Soup, no meat)
  - Calories: 52. Serving size (8 oz) (226 grams)

- Herring - Kippered (Fish)
  - Calories: 87. Serving size (1.5 oz) (42 grams)

- Caviar (Fish Eggs)
  - Calories: 140. Serving size (3.5 oz) (100 grams)

Don'ts:

- Blini (Russian Pancakes)
  - Calories: 358. Serving Size: 3 Large Pancakes (8 oz) (226 grams)

- Pelmini (Ravioli/Dumplings)
  - Calories: 310. Serving Size (8 oz) (226 grams)

- Guriev Porridge
  - Calories: 300. Serving Size (7.6 oz) (216 grams)

- Seledka (Selyodka) Pod Shuboy (Herring Salad w/ layers of Mayo)
  -Calories: 431. Serving Size (11 oz) (316 grams)

- Pierogi (Pastries stuffed w/ Potato Filling)
  - Calories: 220. Serving Size: 4 Pierogi (4 oz) (113 grams)

Belgium

Do's:

- Konijn in geuze (Rabbit in Gueze – a fermented, sour beer)
  -Calories: 300. Serving Size (10 oz) (283 grams)

- Pate (w/ Goose Liver)
  -Calories: 131. Serving Size (1 oz) (28 grams)

- Salade Liégeoise (Green salad)
  - Calories: 35. Serving Size (5.6 oz) (161.0 grams)

- Godiva Chocolate Truffles
  - Calories: 210. Serving Size: 2 Truffles

Don'ts:

- Mosselen-friet (Mussels and Fries)
  -Calories: 894. Serving Size (6.8 oz) (195 grams) +12 Mussels

- Frieten (Large Cut Fries)
  - Calories: 810. Serving Size (6.8 oz) (195 grams)

- Waffles w/ Syrup and Butter
  - Calories: 620. Serving Size (7.5 oz) (214 grams)

German

Do's:

- Frankfurters (Sausage Hot Dog)
  - Calories: 145. Serving Size: 1 Hot Dog (1.83 oz) (52 grams)

- Bratwurst (Scalded Sausage)
  - Calories: 281. Serving Size: 1 Link (3 oz) (85 grams)

- Schnitzel (Breaded Veal Cutlet)
  - Calories: 228. Serving Size (3.5 oz) (100 grams)

- Spätzle (Pasta)
  - Calories: 132. Serving Size (3.5 oz) (100 grams)

- Rye Bread
  - Calories: 73. Serving Size (1 oz) (28.3 grams)

- Sauerkraut
  - Calories: 27. Serving Size (8 oz) (226 grams)

- Horseradish
  - Calories: 7. Serving Size: 1 tbsp (0.5 oz) (15 grams)

Don'ts:

- Strudel (Pastry with a sweet or savory filling)
  - Calories: 560. Serving Size (6.8 oz) (193 grams)

- Black Forest Cake
  - Calories: 479. Serving Size (4.5 oz) (128 grams)

- Frikadellen (Deep Fried Meat Dumplings/Burgers)
  - Calories: 536. Serving Size (7 oz) (200 grams)

- Pretzels
  - Calories: 300. Serving Size (4.25 oz) (120 grams)

Greek

Do's:

- Chicken Souvlaki (Kebab)
  - Calories: 260. Serving Size (5.5 oz) (160 grams)

- Tzatziki (Greek Yogurt Dip)
  - Calories: 30. Serving Size: 2 Tbps (1 oz) (28 grams)

- Horta Vrasta (Leafy Greens)
  - Calories: 34. Serving Size (8 oz) (226 grams)

- Spanakopita (Spinach Pie with Cheese)
  - Calories: 263. Serving Size (5 oz) (145 grams)

- Tyropitakia (Little Cheese Pies)
  - Calories: 182. Serving Size (2 oz) (56 grams)

- Olives
  - Calories: 2 to 40 calories per olive

Don'ts:

- Baklava (Pastry)
  - Calories: 550. Serving Size: (5 oz) (140 grams)

- Saganaki (Fried Greek Cheese)
  - Calories: 484. Serving Size (3 oz) (85 grams)

- Gyro (Sliced Roasted Meat in Pita)
  - Calories: 630. Serving Size: 1 Gyro (14 oz) (400 grams)

Italian

Do's:

- Broccoli Rabe, White Bean & Wheat Fontina Pasta
  - Calories: 444. Serving Size (12 oz) (340 grams)

- Minestrone Soup
  - Calories: 82. Serving Size (8 oz) (226 grams)

- Escarole & Rice Soup with Chicken
  - Calories: 157. Serving Size (8 oz) (226 grams)

- Chicken Cacciatore
  - Calories: 280. Serving Size (7 oz) (197 grams)

- Scallop Piccata on Angel Hair (White wine sauce)
  - Calories: 387. Serving Size (12 oz) (340 grams)

- Gnocchi (No Sauce)
  - Calories: 240. Serving Size (8 oz) (226 grams)

- Lasagna
  - Calories: 320. Serving Size (7 oz) (198 grams)

Don'ts:

- Pasta with Meat Sauce
  - Calories: 425. Serving Size (7.5 oz) (212 grams)

- Tiramisu
  - Calories: 620. Serving Size (7 oz) (200 grams)

- Cannoli
  - Calories: 284. Serving Size (3.5 oz) (100 grams)

- Chicken Parmesan
  - Calories: 693 Serving Size (8 oz) (226 grams)

Spanish

Do's:

- Calamari - Grilled
  - Calories: 75. Serving Size (3 oz) (85 grams)

- Suquet (Tomato Stew w/ Fish)
  - Calories: 272. Serving Size (12 oz) (343 grams)

- Gazpacho (Cold soup)
  - Calories: 46. Serving Size (8 oz) (226 grams)

- Salmorejo (Thick Tomato Soup)
  - Calories: 127. Serving Size (4.1 oz) (119 grams)

- Patatas Bravas (Fried potatoes in a spicy tomato sauce)
  - Calories: 245. Serving Size (8 oz) (226 grams)

Don'ts:

- Cochinillo (Roasted Suckling Pig)
  - Calories: 741. Serving Size (8 oz) (226 grams)

- Albondigas (Meatball Soup in Tomato Sauce)
  - Calories: 400. Serving Size (8 oz) (226 grams)

- Paella
  - Calories: 379. Serving Size (8 oz) (226 grams)

- Tortillas
  - Calories: 362 Serving Size 13" Tortilla (3.95 oz) (112 grams)

- Arroz con leche (rice pudding)
  - Calories: 400. Serving Size (4 oz) (113 grams)

- Churros Con Chocolate (Spanish Dessert)
  - Calories: 553. Serving Size (4 oz) (113 grams)

England

Do's:

- Tea
  - Calories: 2. Serving Size (8 oz) (226 grams)

- Whole wheat toast
  - Calories: 70. Serving Size 1 oz (28.3 grams)

- Natural jams and jellies
  - Calories: from 50 to 56. Serving Size (0.17 oz) (5 grams)

- Tomato soup
  - Calories: 90. Serving Size (4 oz) (113 grams)

- Yorkshire pudding
  - Calories: 125. Serving Size: (1.3 oz) (36 grams)

- Crumpets
  - Calories: 116. Serving Size 1 Crumpet (2 oz) (61 grams)

- Biscuits
  - Calories: 103. Serving Size (1 oz) (28.3 grams)

- Bangers and Mash
  - Calories: 280. Serving Size (7.4 oz) (209 grams)

Don'ts:

- Fried Fish (Cod)
  - Calories: 556. Serving Size (8 oz) (226 grams)

- Chips (French Fries)
  - Calories: 380. Serving Size (4 oz) (117 grams)

- Cadbury candy
  - Calories: 207. Serving Size (1.5 oz) (44 grams)

- Sheppard's pie
  - Calories: 458 Serving Size: (10 oz) (283 grams)

- Rabbit pie
  - Calories: 667. Serving Size (7.8 oz) (221 grams)

French

Do's:

- Frogs Legs
  - Calories: 70. Serving Size (3.5 oz) (100 grams)

- Oysters
  - Calories: 60. Serving Size (8 small oysters) (3.5 oz) (100 grams)

- Black Truffles (Rare and expensive type of Mushrooms)
  - Calories: 20. Serving Size (4 oz) (113 grams)

- French Green Beans
  - Calories: 20. Serving Size (4 oz) (113 grams)

- Beef Daube Provencal
  - Calories: 367. Serving Size (6 oz: Stew, 4 oz: Noodles) (170; 113 grams)

- French Lentil Tomato Soup
  - Calories: 148. Serving Size (9.8 oz) (279 grams)

- Pain au Chocolat
  - Calories: 235. Serving Size (2 oz) (56.0 grams)

- Clafouti (Wild Cherry Dessert)
  - Calories: 150. Serving Size (4.5 oz) (130 grams)

Don'ts:

- Escargot (Snails in Garlic Butter)
  - Calories: 450. Servings Size (3 oz) (85 grams)

- Foie Gras (Duck or Goose Liver)
  - Calories: 460. Serving Size (3.5 oz) (100 grams)

- Duck Cassoulet (Stew)
  - Calories: 548. Serving Size (8 oz) (226 grams)

- Roasted Duck (1/2 Duck w/ Skin)
  - Calories: 1287. Serving Size (13 oz) (382 grams)

- Mocha Cake
  - Calories: 340. Serving Size (3 oz) (86 g)

- Pear Tartlets
  - Calories: 270. Serving Size (3.5 oz) (100 grams)

North American

American

Do's:

- Grilled Chicken (Boneless, No Skin)
  - Calories: 125. Serving Size (4 oz) (113 grams)

- Egg Whites
  - Calories: 47. Serving Size (3.5 oz) (100 grams)

- Fat Free Cheeses
  - Calories: 30. Serving Size: 1 Slice (0.7 oz) (21 grams)

- Popcorn (No Butter, Air Popped)
  - Calories: 30. Serving Size: (8 oz) (226 grams)

- Turkey (No Skin)
  - Calories: 90. Serving Size (3 oz) (85 grams)

- Corn Dogs
  - Calories: 220. Serving Size (3 oz) (85 grams)

- Donuts (Plain)
  - Calories: 185. Serving Size (1.5 oz) (43 grams)

Don'ts:

- Cheese Steak
  - Calories: 740. Serving Size (11.2 oz) (319 grams)

- Fried Chicken Fingers/Crispers
  - Calories: 551. Serving Size (6 oz) (170 grams)

- Cheeseburgers
  - Calories: 1020. Serving Size (10.7 oz) (304 grams)

- Crispy Chicken Wings
  - Calories: 915. Serving Size (14 oz) (409 grams)

- Deep Dish Pizza (4 Cheese)
  - Calories: 640 Serving Size (7.4 oz) (212 grams)

Mexican

Do's:

- Lime Chicken w/ Pineapple Salsa
  - Calories: 177. Serving Size (4 oz: Chicken; 2 oz: Salsa) (113 grams)

- Guacamole (Avocado)
  - Calories: 60 Serving Size (1 oz) (28 grams)

- Seafood Ceviche
  - Calories: 171. Serving size (8 oz) (226 grams)

- Chile Rellenos (Stuffed Peppers)
  - Calories: 174. Serving Size (5.4 oz) (154 grams)

- Huachinango a la Veracruzana (Pacific Red Snapper)
  - Calories: 100. Serving Size (3.5 oz) (100 grams)

- Refried Beans
  - Calories: 237. Serving Size (8 oz) (226 grams)

Don'ts:

- Chicken Quesadillas
  - Calories: 420. Serving Size (5 oz) (141 grams)

- Nachos and Cheese
  - Calories: 1101. Serving Size (40 Nachos; 4 oz: Cheese) (113 grams)

- Tacos – 1 Large
  - Calories: 571. Serving Size (9.2 oz) (260 grams)

- Chimichanga – Beef and Cheese – 1 Large
  - Calories: 484. Serving Size (7 oz) (198 grams)

Canadian

Do's:

- Roast Beef with yorkshire pudding
  - Calories: 533. Serving Size (7.3 oz) (209 grams)

- Fiddlehead greens (fiddleheads, fiddlehead ferns)
  - Calories: 38. Serving Size (3.5 oz) (100 grams)

- Ginger beef, candied and deep fried, with sweet ginger sauce.
  - Calories: 473. Serving Size (9.8 oz) (280 grams)

- Oreilles de Crisse (Deep Fried Pork Rinds)
  - Calories: 174. Serving Size (8 oz) (226 grams)

- Moosehunters (Molasses Cookie)
  - Calories: 122. Serving Size (1 oz) (28 grams)

Don'ts:

- Poutine (French Fries topped w/ Cheese Curds and Gravy)
  - Calories: 950. Serving Size (11.2 oz) (320 grams)

- Nanaimo bar (Dessert w/ Chocolate, Wafer and Vanilla)
  - Calories: 392. Serving Size (3 oz) (85 grams)

- Bumbleberry Pie (Mix of Fruit, Berries and Rhubarb)
  - Calories: 367. Serving Size (4.7 oz) (135 grams)

South American

Brazilian

Do's:

- Feijoada (Pork and Bean Stew)
  - Calories: 310. Serving Size (7.5 oz) (218 grams)

- Churrasco (Beef BBQ)
  - Calories: 239. Serving Size (3 oz) (85 grams)

- Strogonoff de Camarao (Shrimp Stroganoff)
  - Calories: 235. Serving Size (7 oz) (198 grams)

- Frigideira (Seafood Frittata)
  - Calories: 300. Serving Size (7.5) (212 grams)

- Moqueca Com Pirao (Shrimp Stew)
  - Calories: 259. Serving Size (9.1 oz) (260 grams)

- Brazilian Nuts
  - Calories: 185. Serving Size 6-8 Nuts (1 oz) (28 grams)

Don'ts:

- Beijinho (Coconut Truffle Dessert w/ Clove)
  - Calories: 321. Serving Size (3.5 oz) (100 grams)

- Empanadas (Fruit Filled Pastry - Large)
  - Calories: 587. Serving Size (8 oz) (226 grams)

- Empanadas (Meat Stuffed Pastry - Large)
  - Calories: 881. Serving Size (8 oz) (226 grams)

- Cocada (Coconut Candy)
  - Calories: 589. Serving Size (5.2 oz) (147 grams)

Columbian

Do's:

- Pigs feet
  - Calories: 173. Serving Size (3 oz) (85 grams)

- Morcilla (Black Sausage)
  - Calories: 190. Serving Size (2.5 oz) (71.5 grams)

- Bono (Cheese Bread)
  - Calories: 142. Serving Size (1 oz) (30 grams)

- Platanos (Plaintains)
  - Calories: 179. Serving Size (8 oz) (226 grams)

- Sobrebarriga Bogota (Rolled and Filled Flank Steak Boiled in Beer)
  - Calories: 220. Serving Size (3 oz) (85 grams)

- Lulo (Local Fruit)
  - Calories: 40. Serving Size (6 oz) (170 grams)

Don'ts:

- Cerdo y Pollo Tamales (Chicken and Pork Tamales) – Large
  - Calories: 586. Serving Size (15.8 oz) (450 grams)

- Chorizo (Sausage) – 4" Link
  - Calories: 273. Serving Size (2.1 oz) (60 grams)

- Arepas (Cornbread)
  - Calories: 340. Serving Size (6 oz) (170 grams)

- Aguardiente (Sweet Columbian Alcoholic Drink)
  - Calories: 510. Serving Size (6 oz) (170 grams)

Peruvian

Do's :

- Maca (Root Powder)
  - Calories: 30. Serving Size (1.2 oz) (35 grams)

- Chupe de Camarones (Shrimp Chowder/Soup)
  - Calories: 209. Serving Size (9.4 oz) (267 grams)

- Ceviche (Marinated Fish w/ Lime)
  - Calories: 130. Serving Size (8 oz) (226 grams)

- Causa (Cold Layered Potato Salad)
  - Calories: 170. Serving Size (5.5 oz) (155 grams)

Don'ts:

- Suspiro Limeño (Vanilla Custard topped w/ Meringue)
  - Calories: 374. Serving Size: (6.2 oz) (178 grams)

- Aji de Gallina (Spicy Chicken Stew)
  - Calories: 641. Serving Size: (9 oz) (255 grams)

- Anticuchos (Beef Heart Kabobs)
  - Calories: 347. Serving Size (8 oz) (226 grams)

- Papas a la huancaína (Potatoes served on Lettuce w/ Spicy Cheese Sauce)
  - Calories: 489. Serving Size (8 oz) (226 grams)